Retinal Imaging Simplified

Darrin Landry, CRA, OCT-C

Provided as an educational service by

The content of this text represents the independent opinion of the authors and not necessarily that of Genentech. Physicians should consult full prescribing information before prescribing any product.

Publisher: **Bryson Taylor Publishing**
Author: Darrin A. Landry
Cover Design and Layout: Donna Berger
Editor: Patricia Evans

ISBN-13 978-0-9773738-8-8

Library of Congress Control Number   2009906877

First Printing: September 2009

Printed in the United States of America

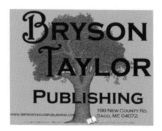

Bryson Taylor Publishing
199 New County Road
Saco ME 04072
207-838-2146
www.brysontaylorpublishing.com
info@brysontaylorpublishing.com

Content

Foreword

As a practicing vitreoretinal specialist over the past decade, I have witnessed not only rapid growth in the field of retinal imaging, but a "changing of the guard". Film photography has been supplanted by complex digital imaging systems. Whereas fluorescein angiography was once the dominant imaging modality, Optical Coherence Tomography (OCT) is now the most commonly utilized mode of retinal imaging influencing critical treatment decisions. Even within the last few years, the field of OCT has dramatically and rapidly changed with improvements in scan resolution and image acquisition.

With the advancement of treatments in vitreoretinal disease over the past decade, imaging of the retina has become an even more invaluable tool to retinal specialists. Imaging guides not only when to intervene, but measures the success of such treatments. Thus, a well-trained, highly skilled ophthalmic photographer is an absolute requirement in today's successful retinal practice. An OCT scan that captures an image a few microns from its intended location will mean the difference between correctly imaging a full thickness macular hole, or incorrectly imaging cystoid macular edema surrounding the hole. This error will lead to unnecessary delays in correct diagnosis and vision loss, an error that a skilled ophthalmic photographer would recognize and not make.

Ophthalmic photographers do not simply arrive on day one of a new job with vast experience ready to work.

While the majority have a background in photography, they often require additional training to understand the different imaging modalities, how to properly image the eye, become familiar with retinal pathology, and how to interact with patients. Ophthalmic photography is truly an art form that one acquires over time.

Landry's book provides groundwork for improving one's imaging skills. I have traveled around the U.S. lecturing with Darrin over the last few years and can attest to his vast knowledge of not only the understanding of the different imaging modalities, but also how to effectively teach an ophthalmic photographer to correctly and efficiently photograph the human eye. Short of having him in your office directly training new staff, this book offers a concise insight into honing the skills of the ophthalmic photographer.

Adam H. Rogers, M.D.
New England Eye Center
Assistant Professor of Ophthalmology
Tufts University School of Medicine
Boston, MA

Introduction

Since 1994, I have traveled internationally teaching ophthalmic imaging to technicians, nurses, photographers and doctors. One common denominator is those who have the ambition and willingness to learn always do well. Ophthalmic imaging is not rocket science; it is an application of basic skills that are easy to learn.

The idea of this book came from years of recommending available reading resources to students that were full of information that was not helpful to their day-to-day practice. What most people needed was a basic handbook, a "how-to" guide that they can use every day to help achieve optimal images, and I believe this book fulfills that need.

Like most ophthalmic photographers, I had to learn the craft on the job, with a camera manual and little in the way of traditional training. This method of training photographers is still the most common, and produces varied results. After gaining an interest in imaging, I pursued a more formal type of education, and have met, and continue to meet great people along the way. Thanks to teachers dedicated to the craft, I was able to advance my knowledge of the field. Some of those people include Michael Coppinger, Johnny Justice, Bob Cavicchi, Jim Gilman and Csaba Martonyi to name a few. Along with organizations like the Ophthalmic Photographers' Society (OPS), the Joint Commission of

Allied Health Personnel in Ophthalmology (JCAHPO) and Eyecare Medical Group, I was given opportunities to further my passion of teaching. Thanks to Deb, Pat Evans and Tim Bennett for their editing expertise and professional contribution.

Therefore, whether you have been behind a camera for years, or are just starting out in the field, *Retinal Imaging Simplified* provides the basics needed to start you on the right course, in hopes you pursue and advance your education in ophthalmic imaging.

Darrin A. Landry

Chapter 1

Fundus Photography

Combining the backbone of science with the finesse of art, fundus photography allows for documentation of ocular posterior segment structures. An understanding of anatomy and disease processes as they apply to ophthalmology is crucial, as well as basic mechanical coordination to operate a fundus camera.

History

The first documented report of a fundus photograph was that of a rabbit fundus, photographed by Dr. Noyes of New York in 1869. [1] Prior to that, only illustrations were used to document the posterior segment, the earliest was in 1853 by A.C. Van Trigt. The first known photograph of a human retina was published in 1886, followed by several other attempts, all of which were of poor quality and revealed almost no detail of the retina. Dimmer and Zeiss Company produced the first fundus images that were of fair quality in 1899. Exposure times were 4-5 seconds, so the images were blurry due to movement. It was not until the use of a carbon arc illuminating light source a few years later that quality images were produced. These were first published in 1907, and later in 1927, after Dimmer's death. After many modifications, Zeiss introduced the first commercially available fundus camera in 1926.

1

Early photography was done by physicians, and it was not until the 1930s that clinics and hospital-based ophthalmologists started employing photographers to capture fundus images. (2) The electronic flash tube was introduced to fundus cameras after the Second World War, allowing for shorter exposure time and paved the way for more wide spread use of fundus photography.

Anatomy of the Fundus Camera

Unlike a common 35mm camera, a fundus camera is a microscope with a camera attached, and operates much like an indirect ophthalmoscope. A ring of illumination is projected out of the camera via the objective lens, through the pupil, reflects off the posterior segment, back through the pupil and through the center of the illumination ring into the fundus camera, to be captured by the attached digital or film camera.

There are a multitude of fundus camera models and brands, but they all serve the same function: to capture light. Once you master the mechanics of one fundus camera, it's like driving different cars; they all do the same thing, the buttons are just in different places.

For general purposes, and because at this time it is one of the most popular brand of camera on the market, we will illustrate the functions of the Topcon TRC 50EX fundus camera. The different parts of the fundus camera are labeled on the following two pages:

1. Eyepiece
2. Camera back
3. Focus knob
4. Angle selection
5. Diopter compensation
6. Astigmatic device
7. Objective lens
8. Internal fixator
9. Pupil setting
10. Filter wheel
11. Light panel
12. Tilt control lock
13. Tilt control lever

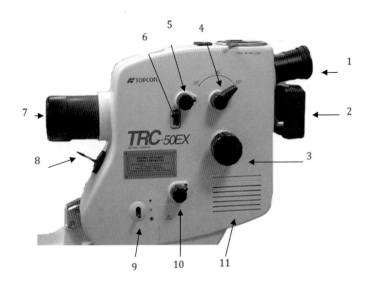

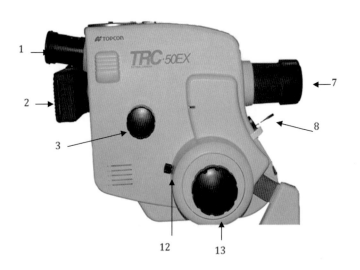

Eyepiece

One of the most important detail of using a fundus camera is to neutralize the user's refractive error. This is done by rotating the eyepiece so the crosshairs seen by the photographer in the eyepiece are sharp, and the process is as follows: the eyepiece should be dialed out to the highest "plus" setting. The photographer then looks through the eyepiece with the illumination turned up and the lens cover on. There will be a crosshair in the center of the user's view that should, at this point, be out of focus. Using a quick clockwise turning motion, move the eyepiece until the crosshairs are in sharp focus. A quick turning motion is needed to avoid the user's accommodation. Once the crosshairs are sharp, check the setting indicated on the eyepiece. Repeat this process until a consistent setting is achieved, and this will be the user's setting on this particular camera **(FIGURE 1)**.

Regardless of how sharp the object appears to the photographer, if the eyepiece is not set correctly the image that is produced will not be sharp. This setting will vary from photographer to photographer, and the numeral settings do not reflect a specific refractive error, they are only reference numbers. It is important to check the sharpness of the crosshairs throughout the day, as pressure from the photographer's brow can move the eyepiece setting.

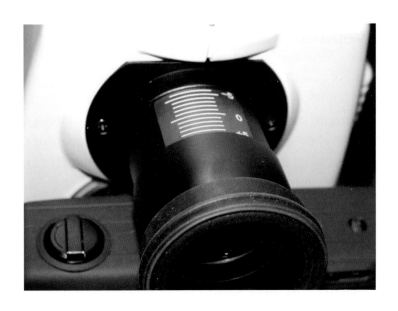

FIGURE 1: The eyepiece on a Topcon fundus camera

Once the reticule on the eyepiece is correct, and the fundus image is sharply focused, it will always be in focus. In other words, if the image becomes less than optimal during the photographic session, it is not as a result of being out of focus, it is more likely to be a result of positioning of the camera or patient artifact.

Camera Back

Most fundus cameras are attached to a digital camera and computer, but are fully capable of film photography. Camera backs vary greatly; some are fully functional 35mm cameras, while others are very basic and functional only on fundus cameras **(FIGURE 2)**. The main disadvantage of using film is not seeing images immediately, as with digital imaging. For this reason, the flash and focus settings are crucial for quality images. To determine the correct flash settings, bracket images by photographing at a reasonable setting, then capture images at flash settings both higher and lower. Once the film is processed, look at the images and determine the correct flash setting.

The process of loading film into the camera backs will vary depending on the model of camera back. Newer backs are relatively easy, not requiring manual winding of the film. All camera backs allow for rewinding the film at any point, and the newer backs will automatically rewind film when the end of the roll is reached.

To ensure images are correctly identified, take a picture of the patient's name or ID number prior to photographing the patient, and include the name slide in the final slide sheet.

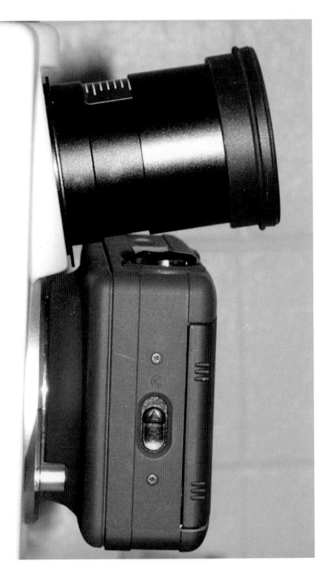

FIGURE 2: Camera back

Focus Knob

Fundus cameras typically have a focus knob on either side of the camera, to accommodate right and left-handed users **(FIGURE 3)**. The focus on fundus cameras can accommodate for a patient's refractive error to a certain point, depending on the camera model. If photographing outside of these parameters, the diopter compensation device must be used. Once an image is in focus, it will stay in focus, regardless of the working distance of the camera. This is important, because if your images start to look out of focus, or blurry, you must look for other causes, such as dry eye or positioning of the camera or patient.

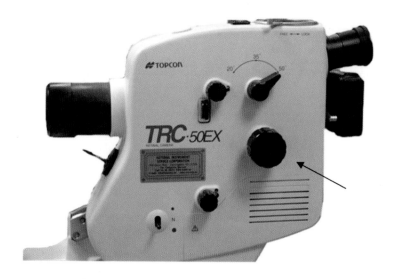

FIGURE 3: Focus knob on a Topcon camera

Angle selection

Originally, commercially available fundus cameras only had a 30-degree setting for images. Modern fundus cameras have a range from 60 degrees to 15 degrees **(FIGURE 4)**, the higher the number of the degree, the wider the magnification. At the higher end of magnification, focusing becomes more sensitive and difficult. As a result, your sharper images may be at a certain magnification, while at other magnifications it may be slightly more difficult to obtain a sharp image.

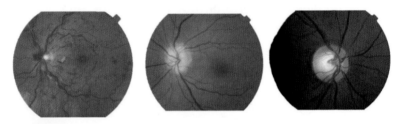

FIGURE 4: Example of 50, 35 and 20 degrees photos

Diopter Compensation

A large percentage of human eyes fall within the range of focus of most fundus cameras. When we encounter a patient who is more hyperopic (farsighted) or myopic (nearsighted), we may need to insert a compensating lens to make up the difference in focusing **(FIGURE 5)**. On the fundus camera, a more "plus" or hyperopic lens is indicated by a **+** sign. This is used to compensate for hyperopic or aphakic patients. Conversely, a more "minus" or myopic lens is indicated by a – sign, and is used for patients with a more myopic eye

The minus setting can also be used to help focus on the anterior aspect of the objective lens, to view artifacts on the objective lens.

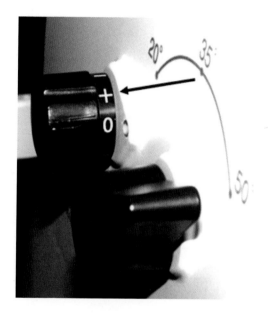

FIGURE 5: The diopter-compensating device on a Topcon camera

Astigmatic Device

On occasion, it is necessary to photograph outside the posterior pole, or in the periphery of the retina. Pathology such as retinal tears, tumors or pigment disruption can occur anywhere in the posterior segment of the eye. When it is required to tilt the camera and have the patient look to an extreme degree, astigmatism is introduced into the image.

11

By angling the camera or movement of the patient's eye to an extreme, the pupil that was once round and accommodating to the round "donut" of light from the camera becomes elliptical, resulting in an astigmatic media. To compensate for this, the astigmatic device can be employed.

On the Topcon camera, there are two diopter settings, *3* and *6*, indicating diopters of astigmatism. Once the lever is pulled out, an axis wheel can be turned to better focus the image and correct for the axis of astigmatism. This device can also be used to correct for a patient who has a high degree of astigmatism in their refractive error as well **(FIGURE 6, 7).**

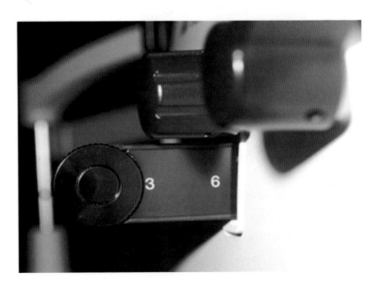

FIGURE 6: The astigmatic correction device on a Topcon camera

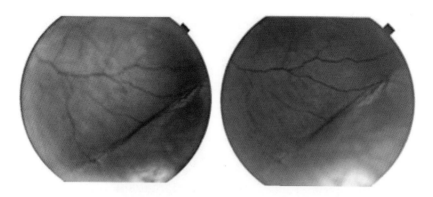

FIGURE 7: Peripheral retina focused with and without the astigmatic correction device

Objective Lens

The front lens of the camera, or objective lens, is an aspheric, convex lens that the light passes through from the camera and back through from the eye. The front of the lens is very soft, and can be damaged quite easily.

Cleaning the objective lens can be a tedious and frustrating exercise, and should be done correctly to avoid any damage to the lens. Some objective lenses are coated, and you should refer to the manufacturer for the proper cleaning solution and method.

Except when actively photographing, it is important to keep the lens cover on at all times, minimizing any scratches or smudges **(FIGURE 8).**

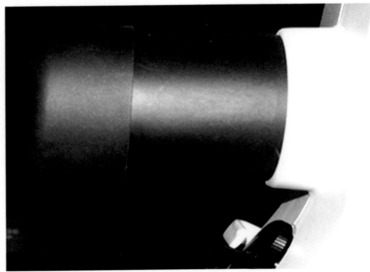

FIGURE 8: The objective lens on a Topcon camera

Internal Fixator

The internal fixator can be used to help patients maintain fixation on a target. This can be used when photographing certain areas of the retina, such as centering of the macula or disc. Left in place, the fixator will appear on the image, although slightly out of focus or even doubled. Once the patient's fixation has been established, quickly remove the internal fixator prior to capturing the image **(FIGURE 9).** This fixator can be left in the image to better mark the location of the fovea as well.

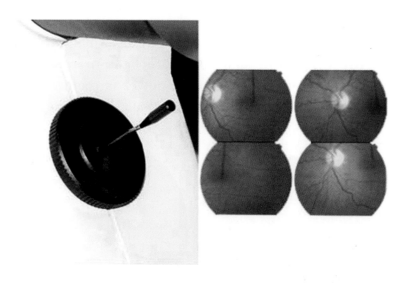

FIGURE 9: The internal fixator on a Topcon camera

External Fixator

This device can be used to accomplish the same results as the internal fixator, without appearing in the final image. It is also useful for patients with diminished vision, and on some fundus cameras can alternate between static and dynamic lights (steady or flashing lights).

Pupil Setting

To obtain an optimal image, a patient's pupil should be dilated to at least 5mm, which allows the "donut" of light to pass completely through the pupil. In a case where that is not possible, the pupil setting on the fundus camera can be changed, decreasing the size of the donut to enable it to pass through smaller pupils **(FIGURE 10)**. By allowing more light to pass back through the camera, less flash power is required. Not reducing the flash power can result in overexposed images.

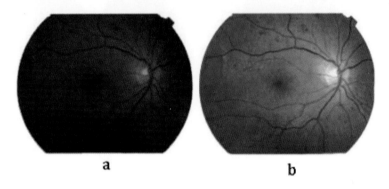

a
b

FIGURE 10: a. photograph through small pupil
b. after using small pupil setting

Filter Wheel

Most fundus cameras come with different filters, usually normal, green and in some cases red. These are used in angiography, but in some cases can be used for fundus photography as well.

White light, or the N filter, allows for normal retinal fundus photography, and in most cameras is clear glass.

By placing the green filter in the light pathway, any red pathology or anatomy in the eye will image black,

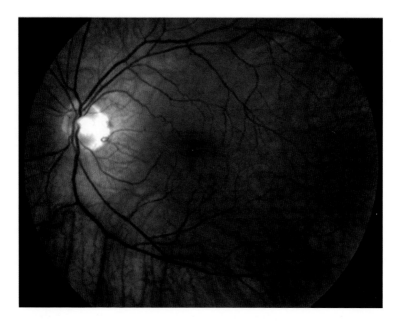

FIGURE 11: A green or red free photo of the retina

providing a better contrast to see small retinal hemorrhages **(FIGURE 11).**

Some fundus cameras come with a red filter, which is in the near infrared wavelength of light. This is used primarily for ICG angiography, and is discussed later in this book.

Light Panel

The fundus camera contains two separate light sources: one to provide illumination to view the fundus, and the other as a flash to capture the image. These two light sources do not affect each other; that is to say an image can be taken with the illumination turned all the way up

17

or completely off, and the resulting images will be identical. It's important to read the manufacturer's manual and know how to change these bulbs. Always unplug the camera and any other electrical or mechanical device associated with the camera prior to taking the side panel off. Consult the manufacturer if you have any questions.

Tilt Control Lever and Lock

To obtain images of the peripheral retina, it may be necessary to change the angle of the camera. By turning the tilt control level, it is possible to angle the camera in every direction, allowing for very peripheral imaging. The lock mechanism prevents the weight of the camera from moving the unit out of place. The lock mechanism can also be used to adjust the amount of torque needed to angle the camera.

Step by step fundus photography

To produce quality images, you must first determine your dominant eye. This is the eye that is used to look through a 35mm camera, or a scope. To determine which eye is dominant, place your hands straight out in front of your face, palms away from you, at arm's length. Form a diamond shape with your hands, touching thumbs and index fingers. Place a distant object in the center of the hole between your hands. Close one eye, then the other. When the object is still in the center of the hole, it will indicate your dominant eye. If the object moves to the side or outside of the hole, it is your non-dominant eye.

After determining your dominant eye, and powering the camera on, the next step is to adjust the reticule on the fundus camera. This is a setting on the eyepiece that eliminates the user's refractive error. Start by turning the reticule until it is at the highest plus (+) setting. Looking through the eyepiece, you will see target "crosshairs" that are suspended in the optical pathway. Quickly turn the reticule until the crosshairs are in sharp focus. Turning too slow can allow for accommodation, and will result in the wrong setting. Repeat this step several times until the setting is the same each time. This will be the correct setting for this eye, on this camera. The setting will vary from camera to camera, even if it is the same model. It is important to check the setting prior to performing any photography, as another photographer may have altered the adjustment. It may be easier to see the crosshairs if a white piece of paper is placed in front of (not touching) the objective lens.

Once the reticule is set, have the patient place their chin in the chinrest and their forehead on the band above. Raise the chin so that the lateral canthus of the patient's eye is aligned with the mark on the side of the headrest. This will allow for proper range of camera movement, and the overall table height can be adjusted to compensate for patient comfort. Too high, and the patient will be unable to reach the forehead rest, or will be uncomfortable during the photographic procedure. Too low and the patient may also be uncomfortable, and eliciting cooperation can be more difficult.

Once the patient is properly positioned, have the patient close their eye. Turn the viewing light up so that it is visible on the patient's eyelid. As you move the camera closer to the patient, use your non-dominant hand on the side of the camera to make gross movements, while using your dominant hand to keep the joystick perpendicular, as this will allow for subtle movements later. Look around the camera at the patient's eyelid and move the camera closer to the patient. As the camera approaches the patient's upper eyelid, a blurry white circle with a black center will start to appear. Move the camera closer until the white circle is in sharp focus, then move slightly closer, causing the circle to be blurry once more. Have the patient open their eyes, and center the white circle on the cornea using the up and down function of the joystick, so the light is within the boundaries of the cornea, and the black circle is within the pupil. This step will position the camera so that it is at the proper working distance, and should complete the majority of the camera movement **(FIGURE 12).**

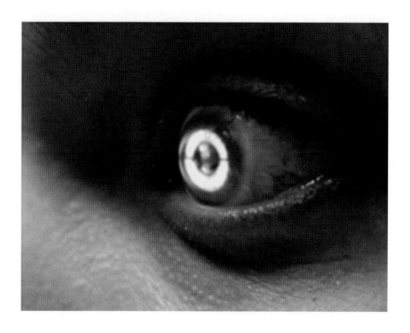

FIGURE 12: Fundus light within the margins of the cornea

Now look through the eyepiece. Subtle movements with the joystick should be all that are necessary at this point. Move the joystick side to side and look for the appearance of white or yellow "crescents" on each side **(FIGURE 13).**

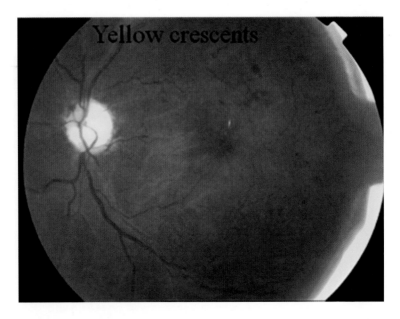

Yellow crescents

FIGURE 13: Crescents may be seen on any side of the image if not centered properly. Crescents are a good indicator that you are at the right working distance, however.

If none are seen, move the camera slightly forward or backward and move side to side once more. When the crescents appear, you are in the correct working distance, and only need to focus the camera. Remember, do not touch or move the focusing adjustment once the image is in focus. Move the camera to the center of the crescents, so that the crescents are just out of view. By subtly moving the camera forward or back, you will notice the saturation of the image change. Too close and the image will appear hazy and white, while too far can result in a ring around the image.

Give the patient something to focus on, such as the internal or external fixation device. Move the device until the patient achieves the fixation necessary for your image.

Find the smallest vessel in the center of your field and turn the focusing knob until you achieve sharp focus. Remember to have the patient blink, as dry eye will result in hazy media. Once the image is centered and focused, capture it by pressing on the shutter control button on the top of the joystick. Occasionally double check your working distance by moving the joystick from side to side to ensure that the crescents are still visible. Capture several images, and bracket the flash; that is change the flash setting one step higher and one step lower than the usual flash setting, to ensure the proper exposure. Over time a standard flash setting will be revealed, and may change with media opacity or amount of pigment in the image.

Move the camera back away from the patient and over to the opposite eye and repeat the steps above.

Artifacts

Obtaining a crisp image can be difficult with the best conditions, but if there are camera, patient or photographer induced artifacts present, it becomes much more difficult and tedious to capture a sharp image.

Camera Artifacts

Dust and smudges are two of the biggest culprits of artifacts on images. The objective lens on the front of the camera is very sensitive to any foreign substance, and keeping the lens cap on will prevent most of these artifacts from forming. Dust can be blown off with a bulb syringe (do not use "canned" or pressurized air, as this can build condensation very quickly, and result in even more problems with the lens). If the objective lens comes in contact with human skin, oil can leave a smudge that interferes with the images **(FIGURE 14)**.

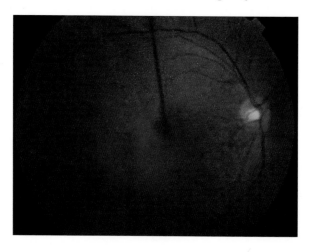

FIGURE 14: Smudge in center of image (Note the internal fixator left in when image taken)

Artifacts that are specific to digital imaging systems run the gamut from electrical interference to foreign objects on the interface between the fundus camera and the digital camera. These can result in black spots or lines

24

on the images, which do not alter when changing the magnification lever. To remedy this, remove the digital camera (most are attached with a "bayonet" type mounting) and again use a bulb syringe to blow the matter away. It is very important not to use pressurized air to clean the lens.

Prevention is the best remedy for most artifacts; only remove the lens cap when capturing images, try to avoid removing the digital camera from the fundus camera, and have preventative maintenance performed on the fundus camera regularly.

Patient Artifacts

Most patient induced artifacts are a result of pathology. Obtaining an image through dry eye, corneal scarring and cataracts is very often difficult. Anything that will prevent the clear passage of light through the cornea and back out again will interfere with the final image **(FIGURE 15).**

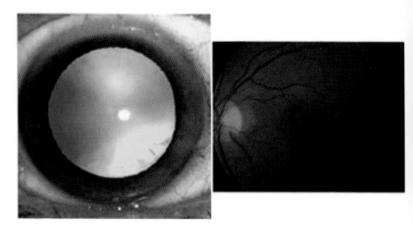

FIGURE 15: Fundus image through a mild cataract. Note how the reduction of light entering the eye results in a desaturated image

Photographer artifacts

Proper technique will result in good images. Most artifacts that appear on images are due to poor alignment of the camera to the patient's eye. Once focus is established, move the joystick slightly up and down and side to side to ensure the best contrast and saturation of the image.

What you see is what you get, so if the camera is misaligned, resulting in a large crescent in one quadrant for instance, simply move the camera in the opposite direction. A camera positioned too close to the patient's eye will result in a blanching, or "white out" of the image **(FIGURE 16)**. Too far away from the eye will result in a ring, or halo around the image **(FIGURE 17)**.

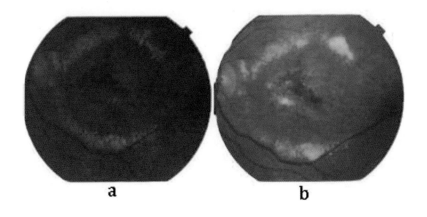

a   b

FIGURE 16:

a. example of an image taken too close to the eye

b. after moving the camera away from the eye

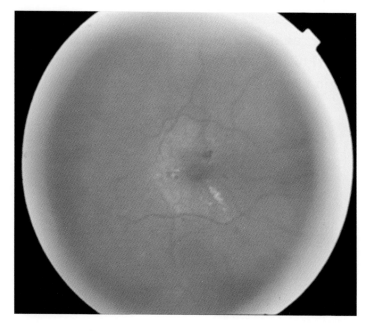

FIGURE 17: Example of an image taken too far from the eye

Common Retinal Diseases

The following pages show examples of common retinal diseases and pathology seen in color fundus photography:

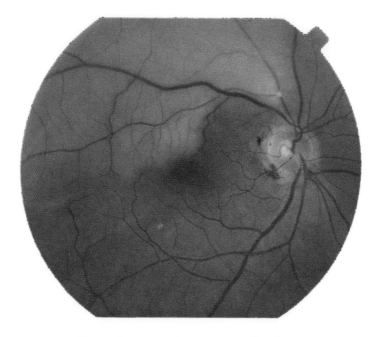

Branch retinal artery occlusion

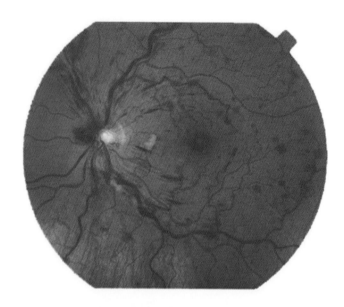

Central retinal vein occlusion

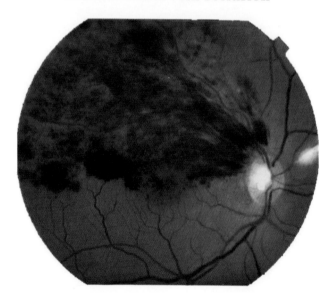

Branch retinal vein occlusion

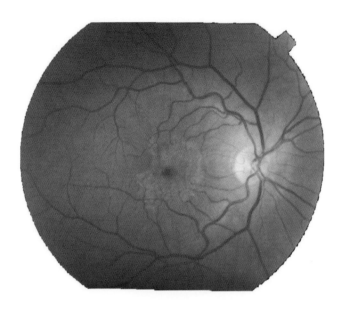

Epiretinal membrane

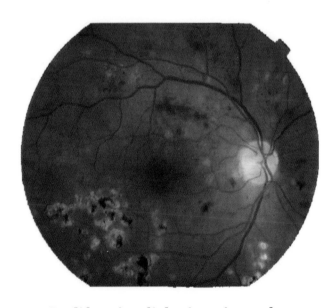

Proliferative diabetic retinopathy

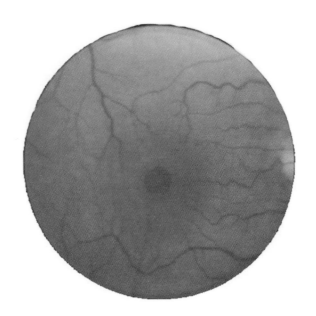

Macular hole

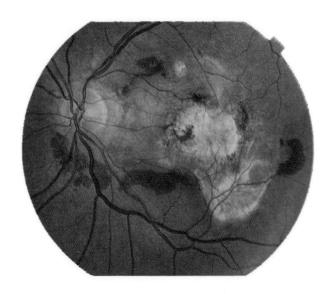

Macular degeneration

Chapter 2

Stereo Photography

A common practice in film fundus photography, stereo photography is a technique that produces two images of the same area of focus, one representing the left eye of the photographer, or viewer, and one representing the right eye. These two images may be viewed with a specific type of glasses or viewer that allow the user to fuse the images together to produce a three dimensional image, which is how the ophthalmologist views retinal structures, either with an indirect ophthalmoscope or at the slit lamp biomicroscope. With the onset of digital imaging, this practice is not as widespread, but the technique is the same.

After learning how to take a fundus image, taking stereo images is relatively easy. The technique is standard, although there are many variations on it that do not produce quality or true stereo photographs.

Producing stereo images requires the photographer to capture one image, then physically move the camera to one side and capture another image. It is important not to change the perpendicular level of the images, and keep them parallel to each other, to avoid distortion of the image. The actual distance moved is slight, about 4 millimeters, but the photographer must use landmarks to ensure proper stereo.

First, obtain the proper working distance and focus of a fundus, and within the boundaries of the "crescents" on the edges of the image **(FIGURE 18a).** Move the joystick to the left, keeping the joystick perpendicular, and not moving the camera either away or toward the patient. This will ensure proper lateral movement of the camera. Immediately you should notice a yellow or white crescent coming into view on the left (your left) of the patient's fundus **(FIGURE 18b).** Continue to move the camera and observe the crescent moving in the opposite direction of your movement, toward the center of your image. Once the crescent reaches the center, it will fade and disappear **(FIGURE 18c).** The image you now see will most likely be less saturated and slightly out of focus **(FIGURE 18d).** Move the camera back towards your right and return to the original position, with the fundus properly centered. Now repeat the above steps, moving to your right. The crescent will now appear on the right (your right) **(FIGURE 18e).** Keep moving the camera to your right and the crescent will move to the center **(FIGURE 18f)** and disappear. You will then observe another image that will be either better or worse than the image you previously viewed on the left side **(FIGURE 18g).** Choose the better image - either through the crescent to the left, or through the crescent to the right. Once you have established the better image, you are prepared to capture the stereo images. Note you may adjust the focus once you pass through the crescent to try to optimize your image.

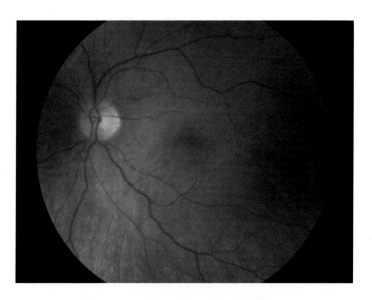

FIGURE 18a: Centered image

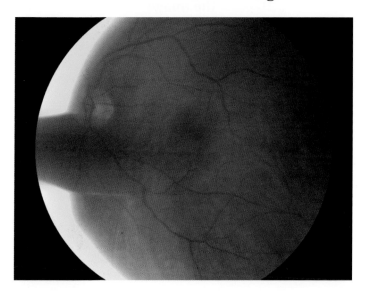

FIGURE 18b: Moving the camera to the left

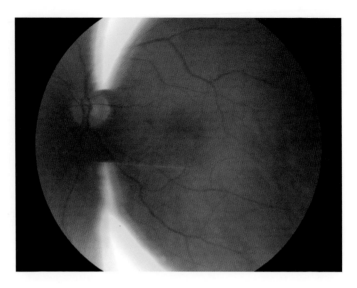

FIGURE 18c: The crescent is passing to the center of the image

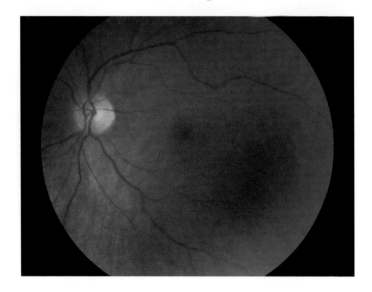

FIGURE 18d: "Through the left crescent" image

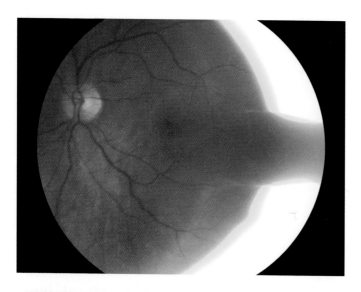

FIGURE 18e: Moving the camera to the right

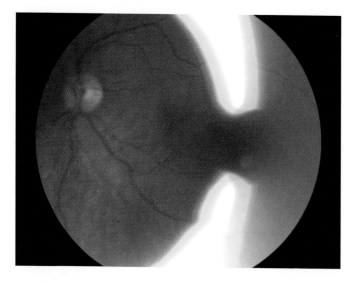

FIGURE 18f: The crescent moving through the center of the image

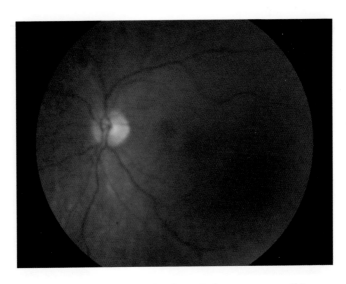

FIGURE 18g: "Through the right crescent" image

Using the above method, you are now presented with three choices of images: **1**. through the left crescent, **2**. centered, and **3**. through the right crescent. The centered image will usually be your best, resulting in that image being one of your stereo "pairs". The decision to use either the left or the right image depends on how well saturated and in focus the images are. In the case presented here, the image "through the crescent" to the left was the better image. Depending on your photographic media and/or digital software, the order of capturing stereo images will differ, but the procedure remains the same. For example, an OIS *(Ophthalmic Imaging Systems)* imaging system will read from right to left. That is, the second image taken will be on the left of the first image taken, and so on. Knowing this, the photographer must always move the camera from right to left. If the "through the crescent" image on the right is better, the sequence will be, first image through the crescent on the right, second image centered (note you are moving the camera from your right to your left). This will ensure proper stereo, while moving the camera in the opposite direction will produce reverse stereo. If, for example, the "through the crescent" image on the left is better, the sequence will be, first image centered, second image through the crescent on the left (note you are still moving the camera from right to left).

Conversely, a Topcon imaging system will read from left to right, so the photographer must move the camera from left to right, with the same philosophy as the above procedure. Consult your manufacturer to ensure you are capturing proper stereo sequence.

35mm slide film sequence essentially doesn't matter, as you can easily move the processed slides to the appropriate place. However, to make both capturing and sorting slides easier, and to establish a standard, try to always capture in the same order. It is important, whether using digital or film, to always evaluate your work.

There are many different types of stereo viewers on the market, and you should try a variety to find the one that works best for you.

Another technique for stereo photography is called differential focusing. This works especially well on any pathology or anatomy that has high elevation or deep features. Examples of this are elevated lesions, optic pits and very deep optic nerve head cupping.

This technique is relatively simple, but should not replace standard stereo photography technique. It still requires two images to produce stereo, but there is no camera movement involved. Once optimal saturation is found, focus the camera on a point of the pathology or anatomy closest to you (that is most anterior), and capture an image **(FIGURE 19a)**. Then, move the focus so that it is now focused on a point of the pathology or anatomy farthest away from you (that is most posterior) and capture the second image **(FIGURE 19b)**. The viewer's brain will fuse these images to produce a stereo image, and in some cases, hyper stereo, or exaggerated stereo. In this case, the actual depth or elevation may not be truly represented; therefore this technique should be avoided.

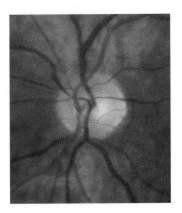 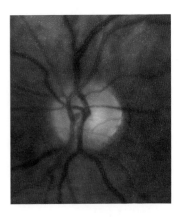

FIGURE 19a &b: Image focused anterior (left) and posterior (right)

Chapter 3

Fluorescein Angiography

Once you master the mechanics of fundus photography, it is a simple step to perform fluorescein angiography. Fluorescein angiography is an invasive photographic procedure that utilizes a contrast dye called sodium fluorescein (NaFl), which is excited and captured by a photographic instrument on either film or digital chip.

History

The fluorescein angiography procedure, sometimes referred to as a "fluorescein", was developed by Dr. Novotny and Dr. Alvis at Indiana University in 1960. After mixing a drop of fluorescein with blood in a tube, they then used a spectrofluorometer to obtain the maximum exciting wavelength and maximum emitting wavelength of fluorescein in the blood. After consulting the Kodak book to find the right filters, Dr. Novotny injected Dr. Alvis with sodium fluorescein and photographed the retinal circulation using a modified Zeiss fundus camera. [3] **(FIGURE 20)** As an interesting side note, they submitted a paper describing the use of fluorescein for retinal circulation, and it was rejected by the *American Journal of Ophthalmology*, but was instead originally published in *Circulation*, a vascular journal. [4] The study protocol Dr. Alvis and Novotny used in

1960, describing a transit, mid and late phase, is the same protocol used in practice today.

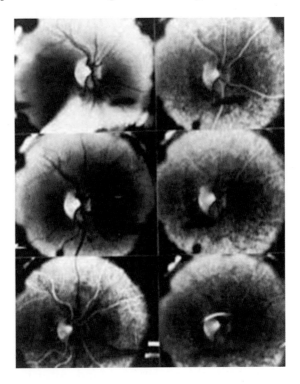

**FIGURE 20: Actual angiogram produced by Dr.
Novotny and Dr. Alvis in 1960.**
(Courtesy of Indiana University)

Fluorescein Dye

Fluorescein was first synthesized by Adolf von Baeyer in 1871. A very common misconception is that fluorescein is a vegetable dye, when in fact its basic components are phthalic anhydride and resorcinol, which when combined produce resorcinolphthalein.

Because of its brilliant color properties, a primary use for fluorescein is as a geological marker that is added to water supplies to be able to identify tributaries, both above and below ground. According to the Merck Index, the primary use of fluorescein is to examine subterranean waters. (5) The Chicago River is dyed to a bright green, using fluorescein, to celebrate St. Patrick's Day. In 1966 environmentalists demanded that the city use a vegetable-based dye to protect the fish in the river, which is perhaps how the mistake is made to term NaFl as a "vegetable dye". Because of the biodegradable nature of fluorescein, it is also used in plumbing to identify leaks, and is used as a biological marker in research, to track and mark certain cells.

Fluorescein has a high PH, from 8.0 to 9.8, and is supplied as a sterile aqueous solution for intravenous injection. Vials typically come in two forms: a 10% mixture in a 5ml vial (100mg/ml) and a 25% mixture in a 2ml vial (250mg/ml) **(FIGURE 21).**

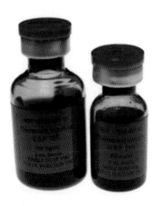

FIGURE 21: 10% and 25% fluorescein vials

The entire vial is used for adults, and child dosage is calculated dependent upon body weight, as follows: the 10% mixture is calculated at 0.035ml (3.5mg) for each pound of body weight, and the 25% mixture is calculated at 0.02ml (5mg) for each pound of body weight. (6)

Filters

In order to visualize fluorescein, it must be excited by a wavelength of light **(FIGURE 22)**. In this case, a blue filter, called an exciter filter, is placed in the pathway of the white light leaving the fundus camera, producing a blue wavelength of 490nm. This wavelength is passed through the cornea, lens and vitreous and excites the molecules of fluorescein in the retinal vasculature. When excited, these molecules then emit a yellow-green fluorescence that is transmitted back to the camera. The extra blue light that is not exciting fluorescein is also transmitted back, and is blocked by another filter in the fundus camera, called a barrier filter, which is in the 520nm wavelength. The only light that then is allowed to pass to the film or digital chip is the fluorescent yellow-green **(FIGURE 23)**. Both the exciter and barrier filter are called interference filters, as they block all light except that at a specific wavelength.

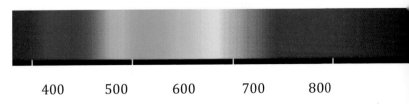

400   500   600   700   800

FIGURE 22: Wavelength of visible light (in nanometers)

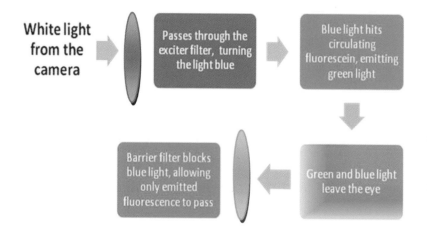

FIGURE 23: Summary of how filters in fluorescein angiography work

Physiological Pathway of the Dye

For ophthalmic purposes, fluorescein is injected in a vein, and then the retinal vessels are photographed in a timed sequence. The injection is commonly done in a vein in the antecubital, in the bend of the elbow, although injection in any vein will produce the desired results.

Once injected, the fluorescein follows the natural circulatory pathway to the heart, then to the lungs, back to the heart, then throughout the arterial system. The "arm to eye" time can vary greatly from patient to patient, but typically the dye reaches the eye approximately 10-20 seconds after injection. Patients with arteriosclerosis, carotid stenosis, diabetes and other vascular diseases may have a delayed appearance of the dye in the eye.

Injection of the dye should be at a rate of 1ml/second. The rate of injection will not influence a patient's reaction to the dye. (7) Only in cases of patients with fragile veins or uncertainty of placement of the needle should this rate be altered.

To better understand how fluorescein presents itself in the eye, and the diseases we are imaging, it is helpful to review the body's circulatory system.

When fluorescein is injected into a vein, it travels to the heart, where it is pumped to the lungs, re-oxygenated, and then pumped back to the heart, then through the arterial system. For the purposes of the retinal circulation, the blood is pumped out of the heart through the ascending aorta, to the carotid arteries, then the ophthalmic artery, which leads to the central retinal artery. The central retinal artery branches off as it comes out of the optic nerve head and encompasses the retina, down to the smaller arterioles, then capillaries, which connect to the venoules that lead to the veins. These veins follow back to the optic nerve head, where they join the central retinal vein, which leads out of the eye.

The choroid, which is the layer beneath the retina, is fed by long and short posterior ciliary arteries, and the rate of perfusion in the choroid is higher than that of the retinal circulation. Consequently, the fluorescein dye first appears in the choroidal circulation, although the first phase of most fluorescein angiograms captured is the retinal arterial phase, as most fundus cameras are not equipped to capture at a high rate of speed, therefore unable to photograph choroidal circulation.

Approximately 10-20 seconds after injection of fluorescein into a vein, the dye can be visualized entering the eye through the central retinal artery. Following normal circulatory patterns, it can then be seen traveling to the arterioles, capillaries, venoules, veins, then exiting from the retina through the central retinal vein. Veins fill in a laminar flow pattern, that is to say they fill from the vessel walls to the middle of the vein, giving it an initial striped appearance during the venous filling phase. The period of time the fluorescein "enters" the eye until it "leaves" is referred to as the transit phase, and takes approximately 10 seconds to complete in a normal adult eye. The fluorescein then travels back to the heart via the venous system, to undertake the same pattern of travel again. Because fluorescein appears in the retinal circulation quickly, it is important to inject in a bolus fashion, as previously mentioned, at a rate of 1 ml/second.

Injection Techniques

It may be helpful for novice angiographers to have a second person administer the injection of fluorescein, allowing for concentration on the photographic procedure. Communication between the photographer and the injector is crucial, and once the injector has established safe placement of the needle, the photographer then directs when the injection starts. The timer must be started when the injection begins, not when it is finished. This will give a true "arm to eye" time, and in some cases can help determine the diagnosis.

It is not always possible to have two people involved in the procedure, and the photographer must also then be the injector. After establishing focus, the photographer then can set up and administer the IV for fluorescein injection. Bring the patient back up into position, check the fundus image to make sure the camera is positioned properly, and then begin the injection. Once injection is complete, typically there is a 10-15 second delay before the dye reaches the retina, so there is time to adjust the camera position and be ready to capture the very early images.

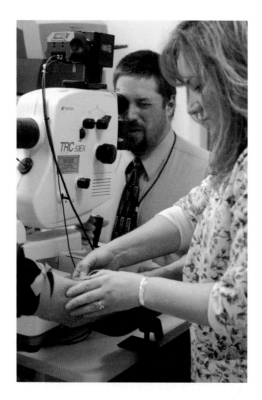

Example of using a separate injector during the procedure

The injector should pay particular attention to the flow of dye into the vein, and watch for infiltration, which is the displacement of dye into the tissue surrounding the vein. If encountered, injection must be stopped immediately. The photographer can proceed as usual, in case dye does actually reach the eye. A small amount of infiltrated dye is usually not an issue, although because of the high Ph of fluorescein, the patient may experience a burning sensation in that area. If a large amount of dye is infiltrated, alert the physician, and place cold packs on the site. In the case of dye infiltration, an injection into another vein is possible.

Intra-arterial injection of the dye, when the dye is injected into an artery instead of a vein, can pose serious problems for the patient. The dye is carried away from the heart to the distal capillaries of the arm, which results in increased pressure and, in most cases, severe pain. Running the arm under very cold water or placing in ice will alleviate some of the pain, and the physician should be alerted immediately. Intra-arterial injections are easily avoided, as the injector should notice more difficulty in depressing the syringe plunger upon injection. Once a sufficient vessel has been found for injection, it is also wise to palpate for a pulse prior to injection.

Complications of Fluorescein

Even in the best of situations, complications can occur. It is important to distinguish between a side effect of the dye and a reaction to the dye.

Side Effects

Although side effects generally are regarded as benign, they are quite common with fluorescein. Most patients will experience a discoloration of their urine, usually a bright yellow that can last for 24-36 hours and in some patients, a yellow or jaundice scleral discoloration can also occur. Patients with lighter skin pigmentations may expect a slight coloration of their skin, from jaundice to a tan-like appearance, usually lasting 24-36 hours. All patients should be advised of any side effect or reaction prior to the injection of the dye.

Reactions

Reactions to fluorescein injections are rare, but the injector and photographer must be prepared to handle any emergency. All angiographic practices must have an arsenal of emergency medication on hand to treat such emergencies, as well as trained staff to administer the medications. There are multiple study results on rates of reactions to fluorescein, and here are some of the results [8]:

- Nausea   2.9% - 15%
- Vomiting   0% - 3.6%
- Urticaria/itching 0% – 0.1%
- Dizziness   0% – 0.8%

As you can see, the most common reaction encountered during fluorescein angiography is nausea. Patients will typically start to experience nausea within the first minute after injection, but may note it later during the procedure. If the patient complains of nausea, stop photographing the patient and have them sit back in the chair and instruct them to slowly inhale through the nose, and exhale through the mouth. Nausea can escalate to vomiting, so watch the patient carefully, and have a wastebasket or emesis basin on hand. Nausea usually comes on fast, is transient, and the patient may experience a fast resolution as well. If the patient vomits, make sure to maintain an open airway and call for help if necessary.

Hives, or urticaria, is another reaction to fluorescein injection, and can lead to more serious issues. Patients will usually note an itching or burning in a particular area of the skin, and hives can be visible almost immediately. Instruct the patient to sit back from the camera and alert the physician. As the onset of hives in this instance is a direct result of the release of histamine, anti-histamine must be delivered, such as Benadryl (Diphenhydramine). This medication should be given as an intramuscular injection to effectively counter the reaction quickly, and should not be given by mouth. Severe hive reactions can result in constriction of the patient's airway, and can be life threatening. Epinephrine is a useful drug to have on hand for emergencies, and is available in a single auto injector, such as an EpiPen ™ (*DEY, LP*). If a patient has had mild hives in the past during angiography, they may be pretreated with an antihistamine prior to the procedure.

More severe reactions include laryngeal edema (swelling of the larynx), bronchospasm (constriction of the muscles in the walls of the bronchioles), syncope (passing out), anaphylaxis (allergic reaction) myocardial infarction and cardiac arrest. The angiographic practice should have a clear plan and the medications to deal with any of these emergencies.

Consent Forms

Not all practices mandate consent forms for fluorescein angiography, but it is a good idea. This shows good intent, from a legal standpoint that the patient was informed about the procedure and any complications that could arise from the procedure. If using consent forms, patients should sign one every time a fluorescein is performed. Documentation of the injection site, amount and dosage of dye used, and any complications should be made in the patient's chart.

Phases of the Angiogram

Remember the rule in the chapter on fundus photography: once your focus is set, leave it alone. This will help during fluorescein angiography, as it is one less thing to worry about. After a red free (or green) image **(FIGURE 24a)** is taken, the dye is injected, and the **transit phase** of the angiogram is as follows:

Choroidal phase is when the dye enters the choroidal circulation. This will appear to the photographer as a light background to the retina **(FIGURE 24b).**

Arterial phase is when the dye enters the eye through the central retinal artery, branching off at the optic nerve head **(FIGURE 24c).**

Early arterial venous phase is when the dye has completely filled all arteries, arterioles and capillaries, and is starting to fill the smaller venoules in a laminar fashion **(FIGURE 24d).**

Arterial venous phase is when all arteries and veins are filled with dye **(FIGURE 24e).**

Once the transit phase is complete, the photographer can then capture an image of the fellow eye. As most reactions to the dye typically take place after 30 seconds of the injection of dye, most of the transit phase can be imaged before any such reaction takes place. The dye is allowed to circulate for a period of time, then more images are captured at a "mid phase" **(FIGURE 24f),** where the dye and background are noticeably more dim, and "late phase" **(FIGURE 24g)** of the angiogram, when the dye and background are very dim. The timing of these phases is dependent upon the physician and can vary widely. Most fluorescein late phase images are captured from 5-10 minutes, as the dye becomes very diluted, and does not emit much fluorescence after 10 minutes.

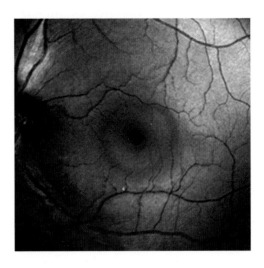

FIGURE 24a: Red free, or green image

FIGURE 24b: Choroidal phase

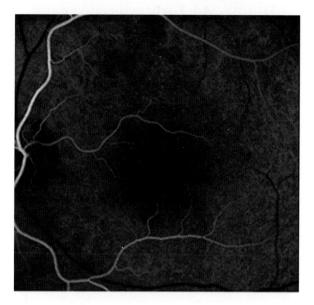

FIGURE 24c: Arterial phase

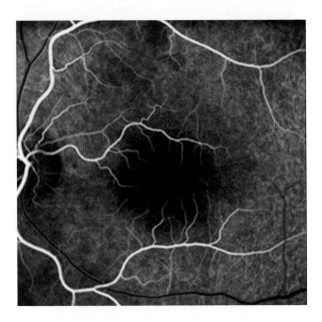

FIGURE 24d: Early arterial-venous

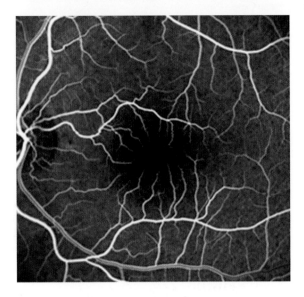

FIGURE 24e: Arterial-venous

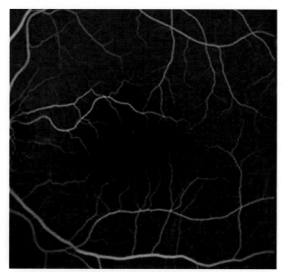

FIGURE 24f: Mid phase

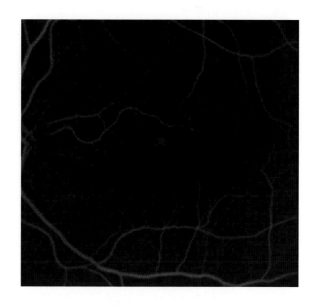

FIGURE 24g: Late phase

It is important to maintain a consistent flash level throughout the angiogram, and not to increase flash as the fluorescence fades in the late stage of the angiogram. In certain instances, increasing flash may create false hyperfluorescence. The same holds true for gain levels in digital imaging, and increasing the gain can also introduce a grainy appearance to your images.

Fluorescence presents in several different ways:

1. Hyperfluorescence This is defined as fluorescence that is brighter than the surrounding normal fluorescence. Typically seen in choroidal neovascularization and microaneurysms **(FIGURE 25)**.
2. Hypofluorescence. This is defined as fluorescence that is less bright than the surrounding normal fluorescence, and can be a result of blockage of the retinal vasculature, as with a retinal hemorrhage or occlusion, or absence of retinal vasculature, such as capillary non-perfusion. **(FIGURE 26)**
3. Autofluorescence. Anatomy or pathology that emits fluorescence without the introduction of a fluorescent dye. This is most commonly seen in optic nerve head drusen and is gaining popularity in AMD imaging. **(FIGURE 27a & 27b)**

4. <u>Psuedofluorescence</u>. This occurs when the filters in the fundus camera have begun to degrade, usually with time, and allow all light to pass through them. If you image a patient with both exciter and barrier filters in place, the image should be black. If you can distinguish anatomy on the image, change your filters **(FIGURE 28)**.

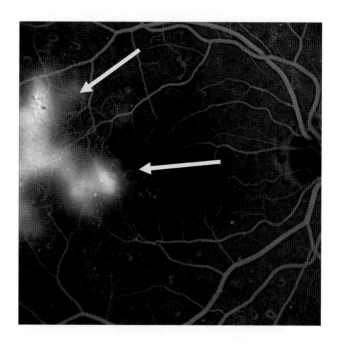

FIGURE 25: Example of hyperfluorescence

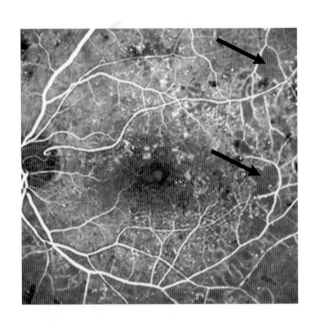

FIGURE 26: Example of hypofluorescence

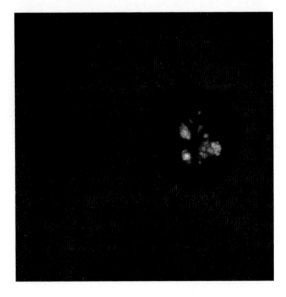

FIGURE 27a: Example of autofluorescence in optic nerve head drusen

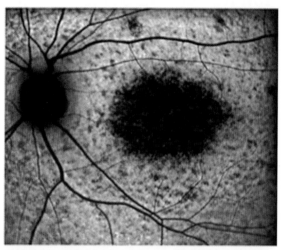

FIGURE 27b: Example of autofluorescence in AMD

**FIGURE 28: Example of pseudofluorescence
secondary to poor filters**

Common Retinal Diseases

The following images are examples of common retinal diseases and pathology seen on fluorescein angiography:

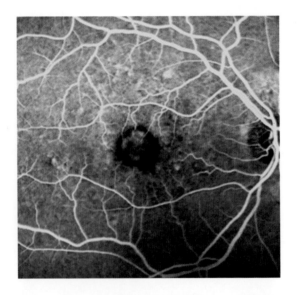

Classic choroidal neovascular membrane

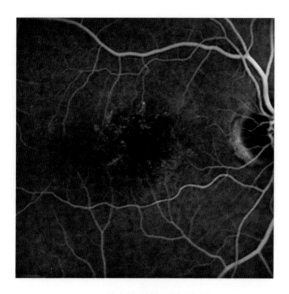

Dry AMD

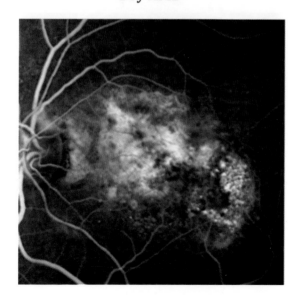

Occult choroidal neovascular membrane

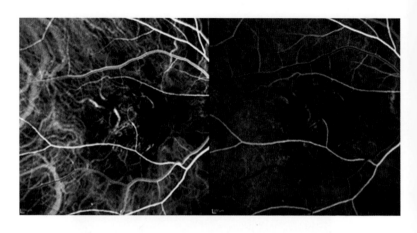

ICG   FA

Simultaneous ICG/fluorescein angiogram in a patient with RAP lesion

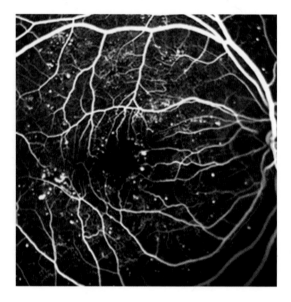

Diabetic retinopathy

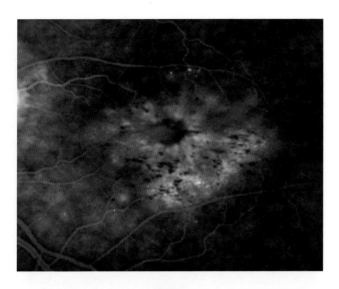

CME

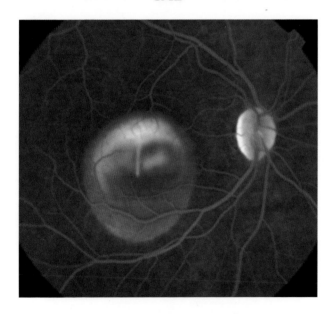

Central serous retinopathy

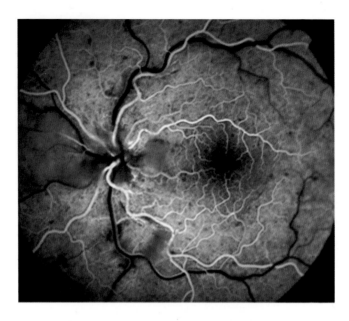

Branch retinal artery occlusion

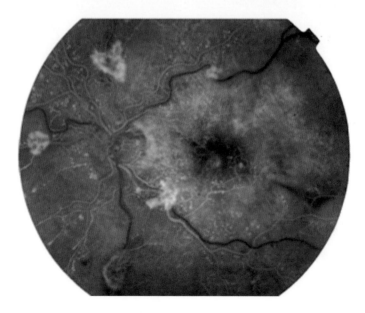

Proliferative diabetic retinopathy

Chapter 4

ICG ANGIOGRAPHY

ICG (Indocyanine Green) is a biological dye used much like fluorescein in respect to injection technique, the use of filters and the mechanics of photography. This dye is used to visualize structures below the level of the retinal pigment epithelium (RPE), namely the choroidal vasculature. This type of angiography is helpful in any disease pathology that involves the choroid, most notably macular degeneration.

Choroidal vessels are naturally fenestrated, that is, they have openings in them that allow for serous fluid leakage. Under the RPE this is not an issue, but if a choroidal vessel breaches Bruch's membrane (the membrane between the RPE and the choroid), the leaking serous fluid will infiltrate the sub retinal space or retinal structures, such as in the case of wet macular degeneration. Fluorescein dye leaks out of these fenestrated choroidal vessels, which is why we see hyperfluorescence in cases of wet AMD. ICG is a larger molecule dye, so it does not leak out of the fenestrated blood vessels, allowing us to visualize the choroidal vessels. The dye is also excited at a different wavelength than fluorescein, at 835nm, so a different exciter filter is used.

This near infrared wavelength of light passes through the RPE and can also penetrate retinal or sub retinal blood in some cases.

ICG dye has been used for cardiac outflow studies, and is secreted in the bile, so the patient usually does not note any side effects of the dye.

Reactions to ICG are very rare, with only 0.5% reporting any nausea, vomiting or lightheadedness. Moderate reactions, such as vasovagal response, have been reported as 0.2%, and more severe reactions, such as anaphylaxis, are recorded in literature at 0.05% (9)

Imaging with ICG and a fundus camera is more labor intensive than fluorescein angiography, as the peak excitation is more intense at the beginning, and then gradually reduces over time. One must use high flash intensity at the very beginning of the ICG angiogram to record any early filling of feeder vessels. These are vessels that "feed" a CNV (choroidal neovascular membrane). The excited dye intensifies quickly, so the operator must be ready to lower the flash to "ride" the wave of excitation. ICG dye has only 4% of the fluorescence of fluorescein, so the flash must be raised during the angiogram, to compensate for the loss of fluorescence over a short period of time. In later images, the gain control of the digital image may need to be adjusted to a higher level, as maximum flash output on a fundus camera may not be enough to capture the dye in the late stage.

ICG is provided in powder form, at 25mg, and must be mixed with aqueous solvent. According to the literature, adults should receive a 5.0 mg dose; therefore, if 5ml of aqueous solvent is used to constitute the dye, 1ml of the mixed dye is injected. However, this formula may vary from practice to practice.

Choroidal vasculature tends not to be as uniform or structured as retinal vasculature and a true "transit" phase of the angiogram will not be evident. At this time, ICG angiography is typically used for identifying feeder vessels, distinguishing RAP or polypoidal choroidopathy and looking for "hotspots" in the choroid. With the advent of scanning laser technology, which allows for more frames per second than a standard fundus camera, ICG angiography is being used more as a standard of care. Scanning laser ophthalmoscopes can capture up to a rate of nine frames per second, which may be viewed in a dynamic, or movie fashion. Individual frames from this "movie" can be viewed by the physician.

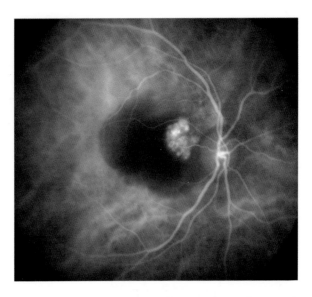

Example of polypoidal choroidopathy in ICG angiography

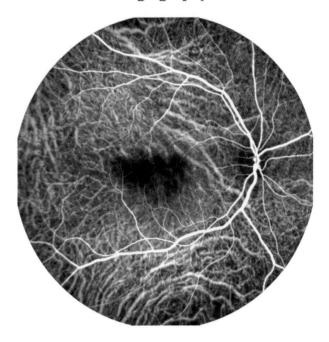

ICG angiogram

Chapter 5

Optical Coherence Tomography (OCT)

First developed in 1991, OCT imaging is not performed with a fundus camera, but is still considered photography- that is, capturing light and producing an image. This revolutionary type of imaging has changed the way most ophthalmic imaging practices operate, and has helped to usher in a different way of looking at the retina and protocols for treating retinal disease.

OCT technology generates a cross sectional image of the retina by measuring the light echo time delay and intensity of the backscattered light. (10) The image produced mimics a pathology cross section of the retinal tissue. The OCT is very similar to ultrasound technology, but uses light waves instead of sound. Sound waves are easily transmitted into tissues, whereas light waves are absorbed into most tissues, and produce scattering of the light. OCT images produce a higher axial resolution, approximately 10 microns, and is about 10-20 times finer than ultrasound imaging. OCT delivers an optical beam of light to the retina, and light either is reflected or scattered back. The OCT then filters out the scattered light and uses the reflected light to help establish the intensity of the image. Only the reflected light is coherent, and an interferometer is used to detect this coherent light. The imaging beam of the

OCT is split into two separate arms– a reference arm (a mirror) and a sample arm (the retina reflected back). During scanning, the reference mirror is moved until the light reflected from the retina and the light reflected from the reference mirror are coherent. The light from both arms are recombined to produce an interference pattern. By scanning the mirror in the reference arm, a reflectivity profile of the sample arm (the retina) can be made. This is the theory of Time Domain OCT, the most common system being the Zeiss Stratus (Carl Zeiss Meditec, Dublin, CA), and images can be produced using a Line Scan or Volumetric Scan, which uses several line scans to measure the volume of the area scanned.

When light is absorbed into tissue, it takes a certain amount of time to reflect back- the denser the tissue, the longer it takes to reflect back. This time delay is measured and used by the OCT to obtain depth and density of the tissue. The OCT software then uses this information to produce a cross sectional image of the retina, assigning false colors to different densities of tissue. The imaging is limited to 1-2mm of tissue, as the amount of light that is detected without scatter is too small. This type of OCT, called Time Domain (TD-OCT) was the first type of OCT used clinically **(FIGURE 29).** More recently, Fourier Domain (FD-OCT), or Spectral Domain (SD-OCT) has been introduced to the market.

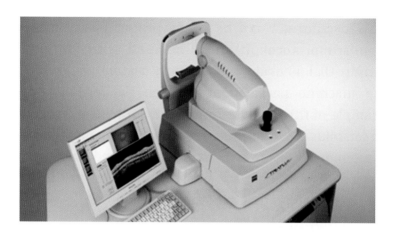

**FIGURE 29: The Zeiss Stratus OCT
(Courtesy of Carl Zeiss Meditec)**

Scan vs. Analysis Protocol

There are multiple options for scanning protocol, but most are a variation of either a line scan or volumetric scan. The line scan allows for a single "snapshot" of the retinal layers, and can provide very useful information. Because most of the retinal diseases imaged require a macular centered scan, it is very important to recognize the anatomy and scan the proper area. Repeatability is crucial in most OCT scans, as patients may be followed and treated per result of the OCT scan. Therefore, a standard protocol must be established within your practice. Patients that have diseases that affect the central vision, such as macular degeneration or a macular hole may not be able to fixate centrally. The OCT operator must be able to recognize this and adjust accordingly. Obtaining a single scan is not good practice, as pathology may lay either outside of the area scanned, or the scan may not be in the proper position. One standard protocol that may be used with the Zeiss Stratus OCT is made by creating a custom scan within the machine parameters that can be repeated. An example of this, using a 7mm line scan with a 7-degree offset, allows a scan to be "anchored" at the midline of the temporal edge of the optic nerve head, and the 7 degree offset will natural cross the fovea in most cases. The steps for creating this scan are as follows:

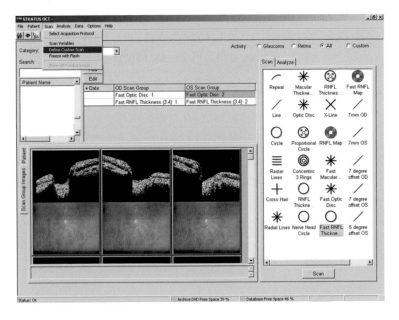

1. Click on *Scan*, then *Define Custom Scan*

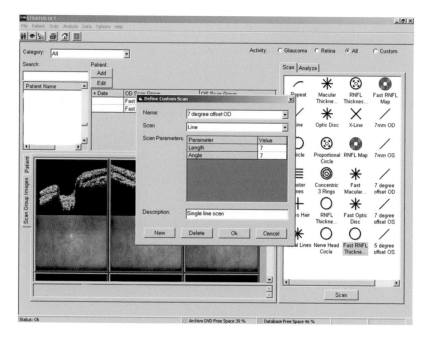

2. Fill in the open window with the above
   information for the right eye (Name, Scan,
   Length and Angle) note the angle is set at 7

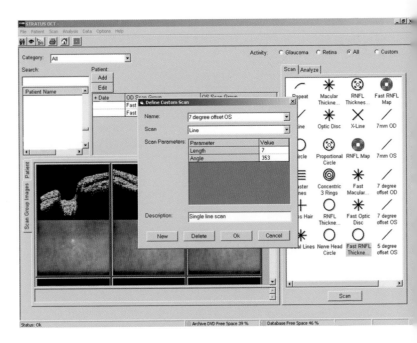

3. Repeat the same steps for the left eye, name the scan 7 degree offset OS (note the angle is set at 353)

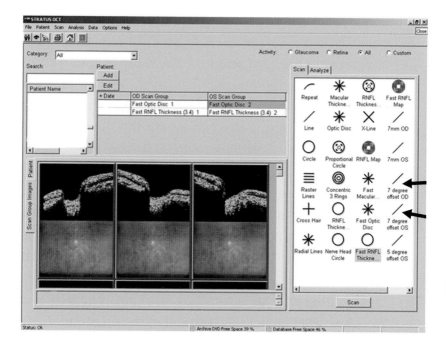

4. Note the new scans are now in the scan
protocol window

Volumetric OCT

Another option for a scan protocol is using the volumetric scans. This scan uses multiple scans, typically in a radial pattern, to produce a measurement of volume in the area scanned. The most common scans used for this is the Macular Thickness, or Fast Macular Thickness Map. The difference between them is the amount of "A" scans used to create the measurement. For the Macular Thickness Map, it is 512, whereas the Fast Macular Map uses 128. To establish an overall measurement of volume in the macula, either for baseline prior to treatment, to follow during treatment, or for use with patients who have difficulty fixating, or blinking, this option can be useful. Because the Macular Thickness Map is a set algorithm of six scans, there are areas between the scan that are not imaged, and therefore interpolation by the software will occur.

Analysis Protocol

Once you have obtained a scan, you must apply an analysis protocol to produce the image. For a line scan, there are many options. In this example of a PED, here are the various images produced after applying analysis protocols:

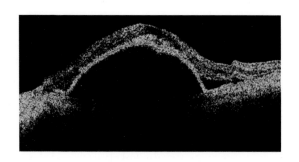

Raw image

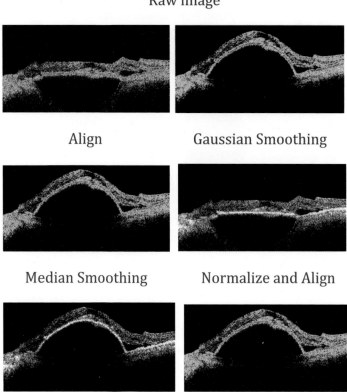

Align   Gaussian Smoothing

Median Smoothing   Normalize and Align

Normalize   Proportional

For the Macular Thickness and Fast Macular Thickness Map, the most commonly used analysis protocol is the Retinal Thickness/Volume Analysis:

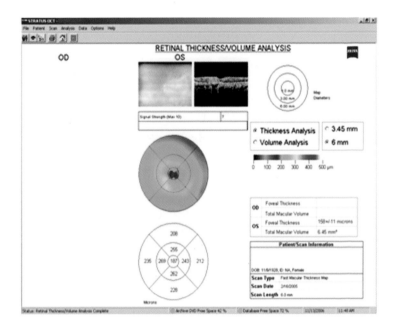

FD and SD OCT

Fourier Domain (FD) and Spectral Domain (SD) OCT are essentially the same thing, and distributes different optical frequencies onto a detector, allowing for the full depth scan to be acquired within a single "scan".

With no movement of the reference arm, this will result in much faster imaging and improved signal to noise ratio than Time Domain technology, and the final image closely resembles a cross section histology slide **(FIGURE 30).**

Simply put, if you think of OCT like A-scans, using light instead of sound, the Spectral Domain technology captures a full A-scan simultaneously, whereas the Time Domain OCT must move the reference arm to capture the A-scan. Without moving parts, the Spectral Domain OCT can capture at a much faster rate, providing more data and resulting in a higher resolution image. For example, Time Domain OCT is capable of 400 A-scans per second, and some Spectral Domain OCT systems can capture 40,000 A-scans per second.

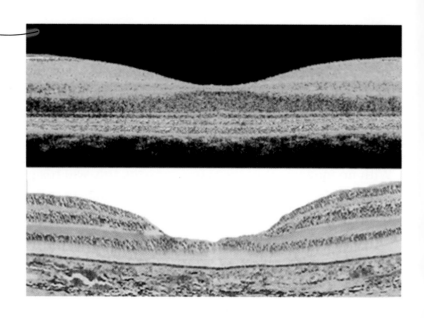

FIGURE 30: A normal SD OCT image (top) compared to a histological slide of a normal retina (bottom) (*courtesy of Theodoros Georgiadis*)

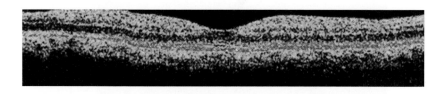

Example of a normal retina using a Line Scan on Time Domain OCT

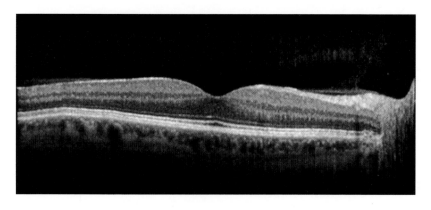

Example of a normal scan using Spectral Domain OCT

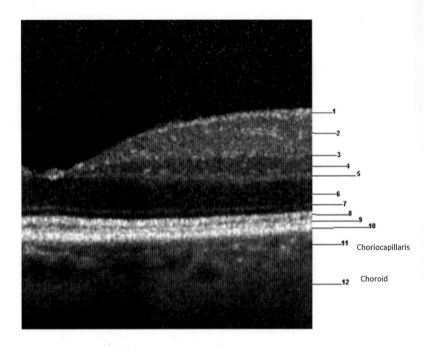

1
2
3
4
5
6
7
8
9
10
11 Choriocapillaris
12 Choroid

Layers of the retina on Spectral Domain OCT

1. RNFL
2. Ganglion cell layer
3. Inner plexiform layer
4. Inner nuclear layer
5. Outer plexiform layer
6. Outer nuclear layer
7. External limiting membrane
8. Interface of the inner & outer segments of the photoreceptor layer
9. Outer segment– RPE interdigitation
10. RPE/Bruch's membrane

Common Retinal Diseases

The following images are examples of common retinal diseases and pathology seen on OCT:

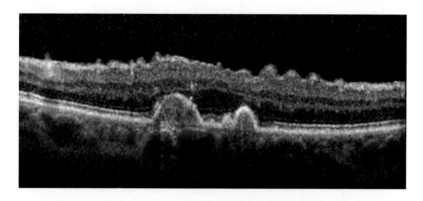

Drusen and dry AMD on Spectral Domain OCT

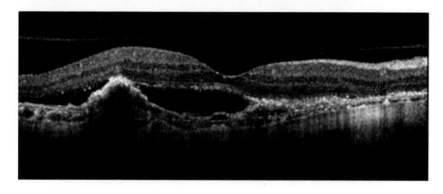

Wet AMD on Spectral Domain OCT

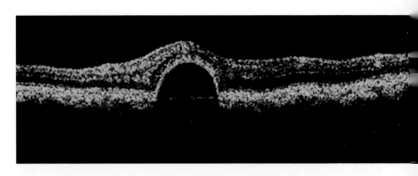

RPE detachment on Time Domain OCT

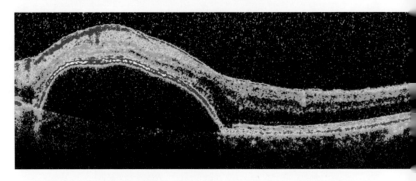

RPE detachment on Spectral Domain OCT

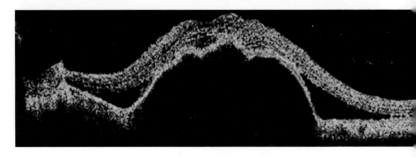

RPE detachment on Time Domain OCT

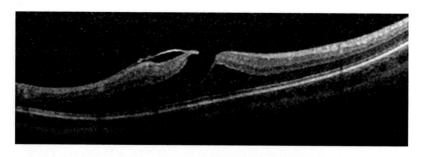

Epiretinal membrane and partial thickness macular hole on Spectral Domain OCT

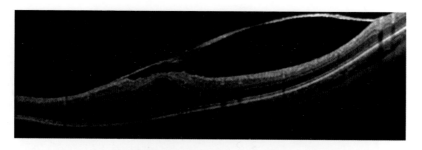

Vitreous traction on Spectral Domain OCT

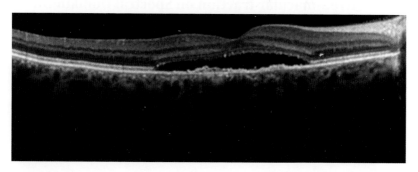

Central serous retinopathy on Spectral Domain OCT

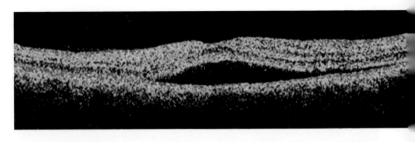

Central serous retinopathy on Time Domain OCT

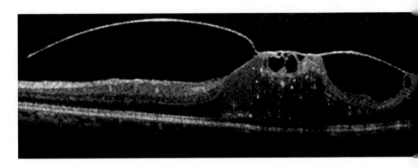

Vitreo-macular traction on Spectral Domain OCT

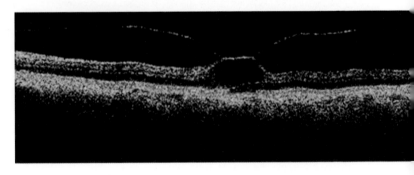

Vitreo-macular traction on Time Domain OCT

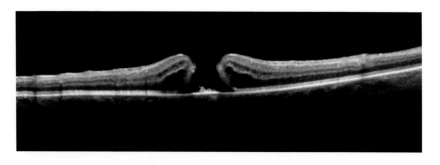

Full thickness macular hole on Spectral Domain OCT

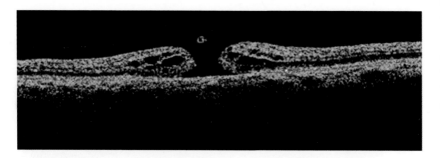

Full thickness macular hole with operculum on Time Domain OCT

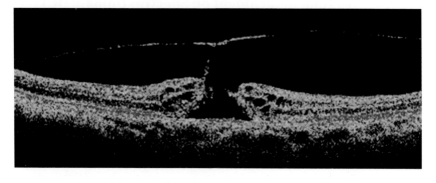

Vitreous traction with full thickness macular hole on Time Domain OCT

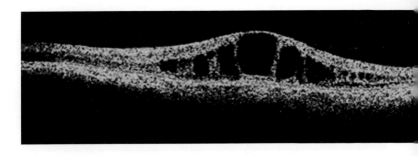

Cystoid macular edema on Time Domain OCT

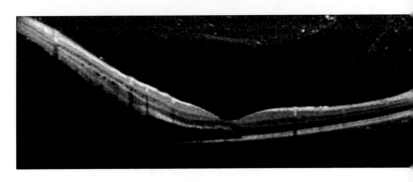

Retinal detachment on Spectral Domain OCT

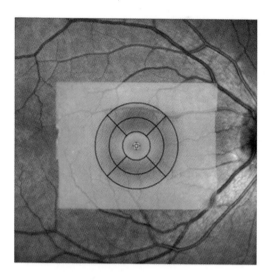

Macular thickness analysis on Spectral Domain OCT

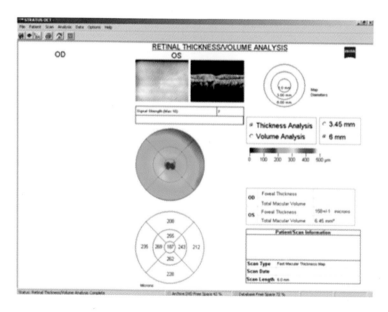

Macular thickness analysis on Time Domain OCT

References

1. Jeffries B.J.: *A question in reference to photographing the interior of the human eye.* Trans American Ophthalmology Soc 6:67, 1869
2. Wong, D: *Textbook of Ophthalmic Photography.* X: 1982
3. Schatz H, Burton TC, Yannuzzi LA, Rabb MF. *Interpretation of Fundus Fluorescein Angiography* St. Louis: C. V. Mosby, 1978
4. Brucker AJ. Yannuzzi LA. Green WR. Shields JA. Jampol LM. Singerman LJ. Tributes to J. Donald M. Gass, M.D. *Retina.* 23(6 Suppl):S2-12, 2003 Dec.
5. Budavari S: *The Merck Index: An Encyclopedia of Chemicals, Drugs and Biologicals* (11th Ed) Rahway, NJ: Merck & Co, 1989; 651.
6. Hub Pharmaceuticals, LLC, Fluorescein Sodium Injection information sheet
7. Larsson PA, Sjunesson C, Injection Speed and Frequency of Adverse Reaction to Fluorescein Angiography, Journal of ESONT2007: 1(3): 22-26
8. Yannuzzi, et al. Ophthalmology 1986; 93(5) 611-617 Fluorescein Angiography Complication Survey

9. Hope-Ross M, Yanuzzi L, Gragoudas, E, et al. Adverse reactions due to indocyanine green. *Ophthalmology* 1994; 101:531

10. Huang D, Swanson EA, Lin CP, Schuman JS, Stinson WG, Chang W, Hee MR, Flotte T, Gregory K, Puliafito CA, et al. Optical coherence tomography.
Science 1991 Nov 22; 254(5035):1178-81

Glossary

This is a brief list of commonly used pertinent words and abbreviations in retinal photography:

AMD   Age related Macular Degeneration

Accommodation   The process by which the eye increases optical power to maintain a clear image (focus) on an object as it draws near the eye. The reticule of the fundus camera helps to eliminate the photographer's accommodation

Angiography   Technique for visualizing and recording location and size of blood vessels

Aphakic   Absence of the crystalline lens

Arterial phase   The phase of an angiogram when the dye has entered the arteries of the eye

Artery   Blood vessel that carries oxygenated blood away from the heart

Artifact   An object that is foreign to its surroundings and usually is not desirable, especially in photography

CRAO   Central Retinal Artery Occlusion

CRVO   Central Retinal Vein Occlusion

CSME   Clinically Significant Macular Edema

CSR   Central Serous Retinopathy

Digital chip   In photography, it is the silicone media on which images are stored

Diopter   Unit of measure that indicates the refractive power of a lens

DME   Diabetic Macular Edema

Drusen   Hyaline deposits on Bruch's membrane, may be an early indicator of AMD

Emmetropic   Having no refractive error

ERM   Epiretinal Membrane

Excitation   The state at which particles emit a fluorescence caused by an excitation source, usually by light

Exposure   The amount of time an aperture stays open to allow light to pass through

External limiting membrane   Layer of the retina between the rods and cones and their nuclei

Fovea   An avascular, 1.5mm depression in the very center of the macula responsible for fine vision

Fundus   A general term applied to the retina and other structures of the posterior pole of the eye

Ganglion cell layer   A layer of the retina that contains the ganglion cells that give rise to optic nerve fibers

Hyperfluorescence   Fluorescence that is more intense than the surrounding fluorescence

Hyperopia   Focusing defect caused by an eye that is shorter than normal (Farsightedness)

Hypofluorescence   Fluorescence that is less intense than the surrounding fluorescence

ICGA   Indocyanine Green Angiography

Infiltration   The introduction of a substance into tissue surrounding a blood vessel

Inner nuclear layer   Retinal layer that is composed of multiple cells

Inner plexiform layer   Retinal layer that contains neural connections between cell axons and ganglion cells

Ischemic   The absence of a blood supply

Macula   Central area of the retina surrounding the fovea

Macular degeneration   Group of conditions describing a deterioration of the macula

Myopia   Focusing defect caused by an eye that is longer than normal (Nearsightedness)

Neurosensory retina   Generalized term applied to the multiple layers of the retina above the RPE

Nevus   Small, flat, usually pigmented benign tumor

NPDR   Non-Proliferative Diabetic Retinopathy

NVD   Neovascularization of the Disc

NVE   Neovascularization Elsewhere

OCT   Optical Coherence Tomography

OD   Oculus Dexter (right eye)

OS   Oculus Sinister (left eye)

OU   Oculi Uterque (both eyes)

Optic disc   The head of the optic nerve as it enters the retina

Outer nuclear layer   Retinal layer that contains the rod and cones nuclei

Outer plexiform layer   Retinal layer where rod and cone axons synapse with bipolar and amacrine dendrites

Parafovea   Denotes the area surrounding the fovea

Paramacula   Denotes the area surrounding the macula

PDR   Proliferative Diabetic Retinopathy

PED   Pigment Epithelial Detachment

pH   Measure of the acidity or alkaline of a solution

Phakia   Refers to an eye that has its natural crystalline lens

Posterior pole   Describes the collective anatomy in the back of the eye; retina, optic disc, etc

Pseudophakic   Refers to an eye that has had an intraocular lens implant replace a crystalline lens

RD   Retinal Detachment

Retina   General term applied to the multiple layers lining the back of the eye that receive light and transmit signals to the brain

Retinopathy   A condition of or involving the retina

RNFL   Retinal Nerve Fiber Layer

Rods   Light sensitive retinal receptor cells responsible for night vision

RPE   Retinal Pigment Epithelium

RPED   Retinal Pigment Epithelial Detachment

Spectrofluorometer   An instrument that measures the level of fluorescence in compounds

SRNVM   Sub Retinal Neovascular Membrane

Stereo photography   Technique that produces two separate images that are viewed together to create a three dimensional image

Transit phase   Phase of an angiogram that indicates the initial viewing of dye in the arteries of the eye and the departure of dye through the venous system

Vascular arcade   Term applied to describe the natural arching of vessels around the macula

Vein   Vessel that carries de-oxygenated blood towards the heart

Venous phase   Phase of an angiogram that indicates dye has filled the venous system of the eye

Vitreous   Transparent, colorless gel that fills two-thirds of the posterior segment of the eye

About the Author

Darrin is no stranger to the medical field. For over 25 years, he has worked in a variety of specialties as a military trained surgical technician.

In 1989, he became an ophthalmic photographer and technician specializing primarily in retina.

He is the president of Bryson Taylor Inc., an ophthalmic consulting company, which he and his wife started in 1999. As a speaker, consultant and trainer, Mr. Landry presents at workshops internationally, is a frequent lecturer and trainer for JCAHPO, OPS, ASORN and the AAO. He is a professional consultant for imaging and pharmaceutical companies and consults regularly to ophthalmology practices internationally.

He is a Certified Retinal Angiographer and an Optical Coherence Tomographer – Certified. He has served   as a   Subject   Matter   Expert   for   the Ophthalmic Photographers' Society Board of Certification, and is a past member of the OPS Board of Education.

With numerous awards for his photography and speaking engagements, Darrin has been published in various medical journals and textbooks including the Journal of Ophthalmic Photography, Insight and Viewpoints.

In his free time, Darrin loves to travel and hike. He has made several medical mission trips to Guatemala where he enjoys photographing the native culture.

He currently resides on the coast of Maine with his wife, children's author Deb Landry, and sons Drew and Cain.

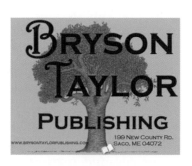

Bryson Taylor Publishing
A subsidiary of Bryson Taylor Inc.
199 New County Road
Saco ME 04072
207-838-2146
www.brysontaylor.com
www.brysontaylorpublishing.com